QUANTITATIVE PHYTOCHEMICAL ANALYSIS ON BITTERS

BY

NWAOGU SEAN NONSO

2014.

INTRODUCTION

Globally, people developed unique indigenous healing traditions adapted and defined by their culture, beliefs and environment, which satisfied the health needs of their communities over centuries (WHO, 2005). Herbal bitters contain blended ingredients in a water or alcohol (tincture) base (Oreagba *et al.,* 2011). Originally, it sold as a digestive aids because of their ability to increase the production of saliva and digestive juices but now has being used for the treatment of various aliment and disease condition(Martins *et al .,* 2010). The increasing widespread use of Traditional Medicine has prompted the World Health Organization to promote the integration of Traditional Medicine and Complementary Alternative Medicine into the national health care systems of some countries and to encourage the development of national policy and regulations as essential indicators of the level of integration of such medicine within a national health care system (WHO, 2011). Bitters contain complex carbohydrates, alkaloids, vitamins and minerals that have antioxidant, antiviral, and antispasmodic properties. These ingredients work together to reduce inflammation, control pain, relax muscles, and improve digestion and elimination (Bodeker and Kronenberg, 2002).

CHAPTER ONE

HERBAL MEDICINE

Herbal medicine in which plants (dried or in extract form) are used as therapeutic substances, is one of a number of practices encompassed by the term "Complementary and Alternative Medicine" (CAM). CAM has gained enormous popularity worldwide over the past 20 years and several studies continue to demonstrate the amazing therapeutic benefits inherent in medicinal plants (Liu *et al.*, 2004; Ekor *et al.*, 2006; Ekor *et al.*, 2010, Al-Attar, 2010; Muralidhar *et al.*, 2009.). It has been estimated that more than 80% of the developing world's population still depends on the complementary and alternative systems of medicine (Bodeker and Kronenberg, 2002). This increase in popularity or interest in alternative/herbal medicine for the prevention and treatment of various illnesses has also brought some concerns and fears over professionalism of practitioners, quality, efficacy and safety of the 'natural' formulations available on the market (Saad *et al.*, 2006; Mohanty *et al.*, 2010). There are general and herb-specific concerns regarding medicinal plants and their ability to produce toxicity and adverse effects. Accidental herbal toxicity occurs not only as a result of a lack of pharmaceutical quality control in harvesting and preparation, but also because herbal remedies are believed to be harmless (Saad *et al.*, 2006). Important additional concerns are a confusing nomenclature, lack of quality control and accurate identification of plants coupled with the fact that there are no governmental regulations on the manufacture, purity, concentration, or labeling claims of herbal remedies and dietary supplements (Sudha *et al.*, 2009). Over the past decade, several newsworthy episodes in developed as well as developing communities indicated adverse effects, sometimes life-threatening, allegedly arising as consequence of taking medicinal plants or traditional medicines from various ethnic groups (Elvin-Lewis, 2001; Chan, 2003; Ekor *et al*, 2006). In some cases, adulteration, inappropriate formulation or lack of understanding of plants, their interactions with other herbs and drugs, contaminants, adulterants; or their inherent toxicity or uses have led to adverse reactions that are sometimes life-threatening or lethal to patients (Abu-Irmaileh and Afifi, 2003; Ernst, 1998; 1999; Fugh-Berman, 2000). Plants may have complex mixtures of terpenes, alkaloids, saponins and other chemicals, increasing the risk of adverse reactions to any one of them or to the additive or synergistic effects of chemical interactions. For example, more than 100 chemicals have been identified in tea tree oil (Carson and Riley, 1995).

Today, alternative therapies have become a significant component of over-the-counter market. Consumers generally view these products as safe and effective alternatives to conventional therapies and most users include these products in their health care providers. Patients do not always comprehend the potential dangers of consuming these products (Martins *et al.*, 2010).

CHINESE HERBAL MEDICINE

Traditional Chinese medicine has been used by Chinese people from ancient times.

Although animal and mineral materials have been used, the primary source of remedies is botanical. Of the more than 12 000 items used by traditional healers, about 500 are in common use (Li, 2000). Botanical products are used only after some kind of processing, which may include, for example, stir-frying or soaking in vinegar or wine. In clinical practice, traditional diagnosis may be followed by the prescription of a complex and often individualized remedy. Traditional Chinese medicine is still in common use in China. More than half the population regularly uses traditional remedies, with the highest prevalence of use in rural areas. About 5000 traditional remedies are available in

China; they account for approximately one fifth of the entire Chinese pharmaceutical market (Li, 2000).

JAPANESE HERBAL MEDICINE

Many herbal remedies found their way from China into the Japanese systems of traditional healing. Herbs native to Japan were classified in the first pharmacopoeia of Japanese traditional medicine in the ninth century (Saito, 2000).

INDIAN HERBAL MEDICINE

Ayurveda is a medical system primarily practiced in India that has been known for nearly 5000 years. It includes diet and herbal remedies, while emphasizing the body, mind and spirit in disease prevention and treatment (Morgan, 2002).

W.H.O GUIDELINES FOR HERBAL MEDICINES

In 1992, the WHO Regional Office for the Western Pacific invited a group of experts to develop criteria and general principles to guide research work on evaluating herbal medicines (WHO, 1993). This group recognized the importance of herbal medicines to the health of many people throughout the world, stating: 'A few herbal medicines have withstood scientific testing, but others are used simply for traditional reasons to protect, restore, or improve health. Most herbal medicines still need to be studied scientifically, although the experience obtained from their traditional use over the years should not be ignored. As there is not enough evidence produced by common scientific approaches to answer questions of safety and efficacy about most of the herbal medicines now in use, the rational use and further development of herbal medicines will be supported by further appropriate scientific studies of these products, and thus the development of criteria for such studies'. The document covered such topics as developing protocols for clinical trials using herbal medicines, evaluating herbal medicine research, guidelines for quality specifications of plant materials and preparations, and guidelines for pharmacodynamic and general pharmacological studies of herbal medicines and for toxicity investigations of herbal medicines. WHO has also issued Guidelines for the Assessment of Herbal Medicines (WHO, 1996). These guidelines defined the basic criteria for the evaluation of quality, safety and efficacy of herbal medicines with the goal of assisting national regulatory authorities, scientific organizations and manufacturers in assessing documentation, submissions and dossiers in respect of such products. It was recommended that such assessments take into account long-term use in the country (over at least several decades), any description in the medical and pharmaceutical literature or similar sources or documentation of knowledge on the application of a herbal medicine, and marketing authorizations for similar products. Although prolonged and apparently uneventful use of a substance usually offers testimony of its safety, investigation of the potential toxicity of naturally occurring substances may reveal previously unsuspected problems. It was also recommended that regulatory authorities have the authority to respond promptly to new information on toxicity by withdrawing or limiting the licenses of registered products containing suspect substances, or by reclassifying the substances to limit their use to medical prescription. The guidelines stressed the need for assessment of efficacy including the determination of pharmacological and clinical effects of the active ingredients and labelling which includes a quantitative list of active ingredient(s), dosage, and contraindications.

THE ROLE OF HERBAL MEDICINE

The pharmacological treatment of disease began long ago with the use of herbs (Schulz *et al.*, 2001). Methods of folk healing throughout the world commonly used herbs as part of their tradition. Some of these traditions are briefly described below providing some examples of the array of important healing practices around the world that used herbs for this purpose.

HERBAL REMEDIES

While there is little to no scientific evidence to back up health claims, some herbalists recommend bitters as a tonic to improve health, especially relating to digestion. According to the Even Star website, bitters can reduce stress, increase and stabilize the appetite and stabilize blood sugar. While bitters will not likely have negative side effects, you should consult your doctor before you begin any health regimen.

BITTERS

Bitters is a liquid that is made of any number of herbs and citrus extracts. This liquid was very popular before Prohibition in the U.S. and was used in the very first cocktails to provide a complex flavour. Before its use in alcoholic drinks, it was sold in drug stores as an herbal remedy, although science has yet to prove its beneficial effects. There are essentially three basic kinds of bitters, aromatic, orange and herbal. Beyond that, there are dozens, if not hundreds of sub-varieties. The name "bitters" derives from the bitter taste the liquid has on its own. The bitters bottle usually has a very small slit or hole at the top to let out only a drop at a time. In recipes, a "dash" of bitters is one drop from the bottle.

ACTIONS AND USES OF AROMATIC BITTERS

These remedies possess the quality called tonic; they invigorate digestion, and promote constructive metamorphosis. They differ from the simple bitters. The simple bitters in contain aromatic constituents, and in being astringent to a greater or less degree, owing to the presence of tannic and galic acids. They are indicated in the same kind of cases as, and under similar conditions to, the simple bitters but they are supposed to have, in addition, some specific properties derived from their volatile and odorous constituents. An example of aromatic bitters is Serpentaria aromatic bitters.

SERPENTARIA AROMATIC BITTERS

Serpentaria: - is occasionally used as a stimulating tonic in typhoid-and typho-malarial fevers. It is more frequently prescribed as a stimulant expectorant in capillary bronchitis and in pneumonia of low grade, when carbonate of ammonia is combined with it. Formerly it was used locally to the throat, as a gargle in diphtheria, and given internally as a stimulant, but it is now very rarely employed in such cases.

Wild-cherry is an excellent stomachic tonic, and may well be used as a substitute for calumba in the class of cases to which the latter is considered especially applicable. It has long been held in great esteem in domestic practice, as a remedy in catarrhal states of the bronchial mucous membrane, and in phthisis. Owing to the prussic acid

(Acidum Hydrocyanicum Hydrocyanic Acid) which its cold infusion contains.

Produced by the reaction between the amygdalin and emulsin? It exercises some influence over cough. That it has any special virtues in the treatment of phthisis is hardly to be credited. The syrup is much used as an ingredient in cough-mixtures.

As regards canella, there has been no proper study of its physiological actions. The success which has, apparently, attended its use in certain hemorrhagic states indicates that canella has properties analogous to

Erigeron: antiseptic, vaso-motor, stimulant, etc. Formerly, it was in considerable repute as a remedy for certain pelvic disorders in women, and was much prescribed in the form of hiera picra (vulgarly hickery pickery), pulvis aloes cum canella. Recently, Dr. Cheron has revived its use, and extols it much as a remedy for menorrhagia and metrorrhagia of chlorosis, for the menorrhagia occurring during pregnancy in weak, lymphatic women, for the menorrhagia of cancer, and for the persistent bleeding after delivery, due to the inefficient involution of the uterus, in some weak subjects. It is also often highly useful in the dysmenorrhoea of congestion, and the amenorrhoea of similar origin. If constipation coexist, the combination with aloes acts well.

FOOD AND AROMATIC BITTERS

Before Prohibition, bitters were sold in drug stores everywhere and were commonly used products. After Prohibition, only a few producers remained. Aromatic bitters can be used in a variety of ways. A few dashes on vanilla ice cream, in coffee or your grapefruit juice adds flavor. Bitters are also included in recipes to add a flavor element to common dishes such as beef goulash, braised pork, chocolate brownies and tacos.

DRINKS AND BITTERS

The most likely place you will see bitters today is on the drink menu of a restaurant serving cocktails from past decades. While there are thousands of cocktail recipes that include bitters, there are a couple of drinks that have traditionally had bitters in their essential makeup. One such drink is an old fashioned, which is whiskey, sugar, bitters and water. Another classic is the Manhattan, a combination of vermouth, rye whiskey and bitters.

HERBAL BITTER

Herbal bitters are a combination of bitter herbs. They contain

Artichoke, dandelion, gentian, blessed thistle, chamomile and other bitter herbs that improve digestion and liver function. Bitters are typically used to aid digestion such as after eating a large or fatty meal or to help ease an upset stomach or nausea. Bitter herbs also act as an appetizer to help stimulate the appetite before eating, usually when needing to gain weight.

Many people only know that herbal bitters are used to cure the hiccups. It's an age old remedy that has been used for many years and always did its job. However, there are many other health benefits of bitters, as noted above, namely their use as digestive bitters to help calm the intestinal tract naturally.

PHARMACOLOGY OF HERBAL BITTERS

Alomo (AL), Paxherbal (PH) and Yoyo 'Cleanser' Bitters (YB), are among herbal preparations that have gained much publicity through the Nigerian news media and have received wide patronage across the various geo-political zones of the country. (Martins *et al.,* 2010).The manufacturers and/or marketers of these herbal preparations have effectively disseminated the acclaimed effectiveness in maintaining overall health and well-being, serve as blood cleansers and effective in the management diverse human ailments, though many of these claims are yet to have scientific backing (Martins *et al.,* 2010). Assessment of the safety and efficacy of herbal medicines is an important issue both for the   health professions and the consumers of these products. The quality as well as the safety criteria for herbal drugs may be based, therefore, on a clear scientific definition of the raw materials used for such preparations (Ogbonnia *et al., 2010).*

MECHANISM OF ACTION OF HERBAL BITTERS

Mechanism and potential uses of Complementary and Alternative Medicine (CAM) therapies is still in its infancy and many studies done to date are scientifically flawed. Further systematic and scientific inquiry into this topic is necessary to validate or refute the clinical claims made for CAM therapies. An understanding of the mechanism of action of CAM therapies allows physicians to counsel effectively on their proper and improper use, prevent adverse drug-drug interactions, and anticipate or appreciate toxicities (Setty and Sigal, 2005).

According to Wei-yang *et al*, (2010) herbal bitters act centrally and peripherally in eliciting their action via the transient receptor potential (TRP) channel (is one type of protein channel), which is distributed widely in the peripheral and central nervous system.

TRP channels have been found in many tissues in the mammals. TRP channels exist not only in the nervous system such as cerebrum, spinal cord and peripheral nerves but also exists in none nervous system such as heart, kidney, testicle, lung, liver, spleen ovary, intestine, prostate, placenta, and blood vessels and so on. Correspondingly, the types of the TRPs channels expression in the cells include nervous cells such as sensory neurons and also none nervous cells such as vascular endotheliocytes, epithelial cells, and smooth cells. It explains TRP channels family extensively to affect the pharmacodynamic effect to most organs and tissues (Liang *et al.,* 2004).

PHYTOCHEMICAL CONSTITUENT OF HERBAL BITTERS

These are pharmacologically active moieties of plant extract used for the production of herbal bitters and are responsible for the pharmacological effect of these drugs.

They include:-

- Alkaloid

- Tannin

- Phlobaphene

- Steroids

- Saponin

- Flavonoids

Alkaloid: Alkaloids are a group of naturally occurring chemical compounds that contain mostly basic nitrogen atoms. This group also includes some related compounds with neutral and even weakly acidic properties. (Manske, 1965). Many alkaloids can be purified from crude extracts by acid-base extraction. Many alkaloids are toxic to other organisms. They often have pharmacological effects and are used as medications, as recreational drugs, or in entheogenic rituals (Saxton, 1973).

Tannin: A tannin is an astringent, bitter plant polyphenolic compound that binds to and precipitates proteins and various other organic compounds including amino acids and alkaloids.(Puupponen et al., 2001). tannin compounds are widely distributed in many species of plants, where they play a role in protection from predation, and perhaps also as pesticides, and in plant growth regulation (Simon, 1993).

Phlobaphene: Phlobaphenes can be defined either as the reddish colored phenolic substances extracted from plant that are alcohol soluble and water insoluble or the reddish colored, water insoluble products that result from treatment of tannin extracts with mineral acids (tanner's red) (Sealy-Fisher and Pizzi, 1992).

Steroid: A steroid is a type of organic compound that contains a characteristic arrangement of four cycloalkane rings that are joined to each other (Moss, 1989).

Saponin: Saponins are a class of chemical compounds, one of many secondary metabolites found in natural sources, with saponins found in particular abundance in various plant species (Xu, 1999). They are amphipathic glycosides grouped, in terms of phenomenology, by the soap-like foaming they produce when shaken in aqueous solutions, and, in terms of structure, by their composition of one or more hydrophilic glycoside moieties combined with a lipophilic triterpene derivative (Francis *et al.*, 2002).

Flavonoids: Flavonoids (or bioflavonoids) are a class of plant secondary metabolites referred to as Vitamin P (probably due to the effect they had on the permeability of vascular capillaries). Flavonoids are widely distributed in plants fulfilling many functions (Spencer and Jeremy, 2008). Flavonoids are the most important plant pigments for flower coloration producing yellow or red/blue pigmentation in petals designed to attract <u>pollinator</u> animals (Cushnie and Lamb, 2005).

USES OF HERBAL BITTERS

The role of bitters in herbal medicine includes the following: -

• It act as appetizers

• It increase secretion of digestive juices

• It offer protection to the gut tissues

• It enhance bile flow

• It improve pancreatic functions

• It act as tonics

• To reduce inflammation

• To control and relax muscle

- To help in the prevention of diabetes and accelerates body repairs, heal wounds and toothache.

COMMON BITTER HERBS USED IN HERBAL BITTERS

The following list contains some ingredients common to bitters.

- Wormwood
- Quinine
- Cloves
- Tumeric
- Saffron
- Angelica root
- Aloe vera

- Myrhh

- Gentian root

- Caraway

- Hops

- Better orange

- Avocado

- Ginger

- Yarrow

- Fennel

- Orange peel

- Dandelion

- Blessed Thistle

- Chamomile

- Artichoke Leaves

(Calixto, 2010)

From the list that the resulting pungent and tangy flavour of the tonic is almost inevitable.

1. **Ginger**: It is used as a stimulant and carminative that is used frequently for Dyspenia, gasteroperesis, show motility symptoms, constipation and colic (Wood,2002).

2. **Bitter orange**: It is refers to as a citrus tree and its fruit and used as a rootstock in groves of sweet orange (while the fruit and leaves are used to make lather and soap. It is used in perfume because of their essential oil, as a stimulant and appetite suppressant (Gange *et al.,* 2000).

3. **Aloe Vera**: Aloe is a genus containing about 800 species of flowering succulent plants (Steven,2010). The gel in the leave can be made into a smooth type of cream that can heal burns such as sunburn. It was also be used on the treatment of cancer, constipation and intestinal ulcer. (Ernist *et al.*, 2002).

4. **Avocado**: Avocado is a tree native to Central Mexico (Chem et al., 2008). It is classified in the flowering plant Lauraceae along with cinnamon.

5. **Angelica Root**: Angelica is unique amongst the Umbelliferae for its pervading aromatic odour, a pleasant perfume entirely different

from <u>fennel</u>, <u>parsley</u>, <u>anise</u>, <u>caraway</u> or <u>chervil</u>. The plant is used as a digestive aid. It is used to flavour <u>liqueurs</u> or <u>aquavits</u> (Gualtiero, (1990)

6. **Caraway**: it is also used to add flavor to <u>cheeses</u> such as <u>bondost</u>, <u>pultost</u>, <u>nokkelost</u> and <u>havarti</u>. The <u>roots</u> may be cooked as a <u>root vegetable</u> like <u>parsnips</u> or carrots. Caraway fruit oil is also used as a fragrance component in <u>soaps</u>, <u>lotions</u>, and <u>perfumes</u>. (Enerst *et al*, 2002).

7. **Gentian Root**: It is used for it remarkable intensely bitter properties residing in the root and every part of the herbage, hence they are

valuable tonic medicines. The <u>medicinal</u> parts are the dried, underground parts of the plant and the fresh, above ground parts (Struwe and Albert, 2002).

8. **Yarrow**: Long ago, yarrow was used during the Roman times to heal wounds. It's still used effectively today to help stop bleeding. Yarrow, a mildly bitter herb, also helps resolve stomach pains and muscle spasms.

9. **Fennel**: There are many benefits to ingesting fennel herb. Most notably is its ability to combat anxiety, depression, and respiratory congestion as well as its benefits for the digestive system.

Fennel also works hand in hand with the fight against cancer, as those who are going through chemotherapy can take fennel afterwards to help rebuild their digestive system.

10. Orange Peel: One of the most popular ingredients in herbal Bitters is orange peel. It has been used for years to work as an anti-inflammatory regimen and curbs issues with digestion. However, orange peel is not just used for digestion. It is also a remedy for lowering blood pressure and bad cholesterol levels.

11. Dandelion: Probably one of the most overlooked bitter herbs on the market is dandelion. Even though it is known as a bitter herb, some societies still consider it to be just a weed. However, there are many health benefits to dandelion that include fighting off bacterial infections, acne, arthritis, high blood pressure, and even PMS.

12. Chamomile: Digestive bitters are extremely useful to give you a healthier body, but chamomile has additional advantages. This mildly bitter herb dates back as far as Roman times as an aid for digestive issues. However, we now use chamomile for a host of reasons. Most notably they sooth colds, reduce gum inflammation, or even to combat diaper rash or chicken pox.

13. Blessed Thistle: If by chance you're suffering from gas issues after a meal, blessed thistle is known to control and reduce it. Then again, this bitter herb is known for helping us in several areas that include healing wounds, skin ulcers, acne, and many others. Whether you are having digestive issues or simply need something to eliminate bacteria, blessed thistle is the primary herb to use.

14. Artichoke leaves: Even though most of the bitter herbs are geared towards the digestive tract, artichoke leaves have additional benefits. They help lower your bad cholesterol, combat kidney disease, help calm and eliminate diarrhea, vomiting, nausea, and help to control heartburn, bloating, and abdominal pain. There are many other advantages as well, but these are the most popular.

HOW TO USE HERBAL BITTERS

Most bitter herbs can be used in teas or tinctures. Many are also available in capsule form. There are also some wonderful herbal bitters combinations that can be taken diluted in water.

BITTER HERBS

Bitter herbs are one of herbal medicine's great contributions to human health. Quite simply, this category contains herbs that have a bitter taste, ranging from mildly bitter yarrow to fiercely bitter rue. Absinthin, a constituent found in wormwood, is so bitter it can be tasted even at dilutions of 1 part in 30,000 parts of water. The strong flavour is often attributed to a bitter principle, which can be a volatile oil, an alkaloid, an iridoid, or a sesquiterpene. Following stimulation of the bitter receptors, located at the back of the tongue, a range of physiological responses occurs. Specific taste buds transmit the taste of bitterness to the central nervous system, triggering a number of reflexes. These reflexes have important ramifications, all of value to the digestive process and general health.

The stimulation of the flow of digestive juices from the exocrine glands of the mouth, stomach, pancreas, duodenum, and liver aid in good digestion as well as helping a range of conditions caused by inefficient or allergy-distorted digestion. The flow of digestive juices triggers a stimulation of appetite. This is helpful in convalescence as well as in cases of appetite reduction. A range of liver activities is stimulated, including increased bile production and the release of bile from the gallbladder. A very mild stimulation of the endocrine glands occurs, producing insulin and glucagon secretions from the islets of Langerhans in the pancreas. Diabetics need to use bitters cautiously, as these herbs can change the blood sugar balance. In the hands of a skilled practitioner, however, bitter remedies can play a role in the treatment of non-insulin dependent diabetes.

Bitter remedies can trigger subtle psychological effects, even acting as mild antidepressants. For example, bitters can help lift the spirits in cases of post-viral-infection depression. The central reflex stimulates peristalsis, an action that moves wastes through the intestines through a series of muscular contractions.

Bitter remedies also stimulate the gut wall's self-repair mechanisms.

Some common herbal bitters are: -

- Barberry (pictured)

- Boneset

- Chamomile

- Dandelion

- Gentian

- Goldenseal

- Hop

- Horehound

- Mugwort

- Rue

- Southernwood

- Tansy

- Wormwood

- Yarrow

USES OF BITTERS

Bitters are a diverse group of chemicals compounds that share the common characteristic of a bitter taste. Bitters can be used to strengthen and improve the whole digestive system in the body as well as the nervous system. Bitters also act to increase the vital energy centers in the body. Because they have such a broad effect on the entire physiology, tone and function of the body bitters are a principle that can be used to treat the body as a whole. The beneficial effects of bitters go beyond digestive hormone activity. Bitter stimulation can often shift a condition or illness that does not appear to have anything to do with the digestive process. The bitter principal acts to increase self-healing and resistance in many ways.

THE BITTER TASTE

To be effective bitters must be tasted on the taste buds of the tongue where they stimulate the bitter taste buds on the tongue and thus increase salivation. This stimulates the gastric reflex to cause digestive juices to be secreted. There is increased flow of digestive juices from the pancreas, duodenum, and liver that results in better assimilation of nutrients and less undigested food being passed through the digestive tract. This is of benefit to problems that have their basis in inefficient or allergy distorted digestion.

THE BITTERING AGENT

This will be the ingredient that will make your bitters, well, bitter.

Common ingredients are gentian, quassia or even wormwood (famous as

An ingredient in absinthe). These flora are usually extremely bitter, and a little will go a long way.

THE FLAVOUR

This is where you have your chance to show off your creativity. Simple bitters will have one flavour, such as orange or peach or grapefruit. But the sky is the limit when it comes to bitters. Obviously more ingredients will add more complexity to your bitters, just make sure that they play together and remember, sometimes simple one and two flavour bitters are better.

THE SOLUTION

Most bitters are kept in alcohol, but you can make non-alcoholic bitters if you really wanted (they will have a very short shelf life). Try to find the highest proof alcohol you can get your hands on (50% above is best, don't go over 60% above), as this seems to extract more flavour from my herbs and spices as well as give the final product an indefiniteshelf life (alcohol is a preservative after all). For lighter bitters you may use a high-proof vodka or gin as the solution, while rum, whiskey and brandy are the spirits that you look to when creating heavier, darker bitters. Now, most bitter recipes you will see that they have you throw all of the ingredients in a jar and wait a period of time (anywhere from a couple of days to a couple of months) after which you will filter and bottle your final product.

Different ingredients will release their respective flavours at different speeds and so to circumvent the probability of one ingredient's flavour overpowering the batch, give each flavour profile its own vessel. For example, if you were to do a batch of simple orange bitters, you would start with two jars of alcohol, one with gentian and the other with orange peel. After a period of one week, you would strain out the gentian and after three weeks, you would strain out the orange peel. You would then slowly add the gentian mixture to the orange peel until the desired level of bitterness was reached. It is with this blending technique that you can ensure that you will never ruin a batch of bitters beyond repair, as an over powering flavours can be adjusted by increasing the other flavor components of the batch. As for filtering, you can use coffee filters but it is extremely time consuming and laborious. You switch over to a Buchner funnel with a hand vacuum, but even this can be a little too much work.

THE VARIOUS ROLES OF BITTERS

Bitters act to increase or stabilize the appetite. In general, there is a stimulation of the appetite which is important in conditions of convalescence and where there is otherwise a reduction of appetite.

Bitters do not seem to increase appetite in a digestively healthy person, rather a more healthful balance in the appetite develops. The body acquires more taste for healthy foods and less taste for unhealthy foods.

When bitters activate the gastric secretion of hydrochloric acid and other digestive enzymes, the nerve tone of the muscles of the entire digestive tract improves. Blood circulation improves and the body can assimilate foods, absorb nutrients, and eliminate wastes more efficiently. In a broader way, this improvement in blood circulation affects the healthy activity of the heart and circulation in general.

CLEANSING AND DETOXIFICATION

Bitters stimulate the liver to do a more effective cleansing and detoxifying job and prompt the gallbladder to make bile. The production of bile helps metabolize fats and keeps elimination moving smoothly. Bitters also produce a diuretic and hepatic effect in the body. This has value when working with any condition that has origins in a sluggish or overworked liver.

1. STABILIZING BLOOD SUGAR

Bitters produce a regulatory effect on the secretion of the pancreas of the hormones that regulate blood sugar, insulin, and glucagon. This can be of benefit in stabilizing insulin levels and modulating blood sugar swings. Diabetics should be careful when taking bitters because bitters may upset their blood sugar balance.

2. REDUCING STRESS

Bitters can also be supportive in reducing stress and anxiety and regenerating the nervous system. When bitters work to strengthen digestion this activates the parasympathetic branch of the autonomic nervous system and induces a more relaxed state in the body. Bitters can be useful with those who are overextended and stressed out. Bitters produce subtle, beneficial psychological effects. In some cases they can produce a marked antidepressant effect and a "generally tonic effect upon consciousness."

3. INCREASING IMMUNE RESPONSES

Some bitter herbs such as Gentian can modulate the gut associated immune responses. In some therapeutic circles bitters are indicated for treatment of those recovering from infectious diseases including viral conditions such as chronic fatigue syndrome. Some clinical tests have shown that bitters can decrease levels of sIgA antibodies and reduce or eliminate symptoms in those with inflammatory bowel disease. Bitters may help repair gut wall damage through stimulating self-repair mechanisms.

WHO SHOULD USE BITTERS?

Bitters are indicated when there is digestive weakness. Digestive weakness is often associated with an infectious disease that depletes the vital energy of the body. Digestive weakness and decreased vitality both reduce the assimilation of nutrients and the elimination of wastes resulting in a spiraling effect of depletion in the body. Stress can deplete vital energy which disrupts digestion and this further decreases the body's vital energy.

Bitters can also be useful for those who have an over reliance on mental energy that can result in physical exhaustion.

Bitters are indicated for use in: -

- Poor fat digestion

- Poor protein digestion

- Weakness due to chronic illness especially with a bacterial or viral

- Infection

- Loss of energy and vitality

- Painful digestion

- Intestinal cramps

- Excessive gas

- Irritable bowel syndrome

- Poor appetite

- Anemia

- Excessive craving for sweets, fats, and carbohydrates

- Immune disorders where nutritional deficiency is present

- Digestive weakness due to mental overwork and lack of exercise.

WHICH HERBS ARE BITTERS?

Important bitter herbs include: -

Peppermint, Calendula, Dandelion, Artichoke leaf, Blessed Thistle, Angelica, Motherwort, Wormwood, Bitter orange peel, Lemon peel, Gentian root, Centaury root, Mugwort, Goldenseal, Cascara Sagrada, Devils Claw,

Tarragon, Hops, Boneset, Barberry, Chamomile, Yarrow, Horehound, and Tansy.

Bitters range in effect from mild bitters like Chamomile to intense bitters like Wormwood or Gentian. The whole bitters class of herbs has a variable therapeutic margin. The more mild the bitter the greater the therapeutic range and the more intense the bitter the more restrictive the range. Intense bitters like Wormwood, Tansy, and Rue have a low therapeutic margin and need to be used with care. Absinthinn found in Artemisias such as Wormwood is so bitter it can be tasted at a dilution of 1:30,000. A mild bitter like Chamomile has a very wide therapeutic margin and can be used in much greater quantities for a larger population. In general, though bitters are taken in small quantities at meals and are not usually consumed by the cupfuls throughout the day.

How to take your Bitters

Bitters extract well into hot water and alcohol. Bitters may be combined with flavourful herbs such as Licorice, Orange peel, Lemon peel, Cardomen to give a better tasting remedy. Some bitters are destroyed by heat and most bitters are taken in alcohol preparations. To gain their full effectiveness bitters should be taken over time. Some effect may be seen immediately, but their fullest benefit in the body is achieved when they are taken over weeks and months.

Bitters are usually taken 15 to 30 minutes before the meal or just after the meal. If too great a dose is taken symptoms may worsen. If that is the case lower the dose and gradually build up as the body gets stronger.

PAXHERBAL BITTERS

A Paxherbal bitter is an organic medicine in the class of bitters. It is a tincture of different herbal ingredients that promotes blood circulation, prevents kidney stone, helps in digestion, and activates bite flow, increase immunity of the body against bacterial and fungal infections. It helps in prevention of diabetes and accelerates body repairs, heal wounds and toothaches (Steven, 2010).

COMPOSITION OF PAXHERBAL BITTERS

It is composed of the following main ingredients like Lemon grass, Aloe vera, Rawolfia vomitoria, Sida acuta, Gongronema latifolium, Â Ginger, Xylopia aethiopica,

Vernonia amygdalina, Tridax procumbens with an active ingredients of Glycosides, Lycopenes, Aliphatic phenols, Glycoflavones, Carotenoids, Saponins, Tannins, Quinine and Alkaloids.

PHARMACOKINETICS

Paxherbal Bitters (PB) rapidly and completely absorbed from the gastro-intestinal tract after oral administration with high plasma level for few minutes of administration, although PB can also be used for topical applications. However, the ultimate course of the action of PB for oral administration is evidenced by absorption of the phytochemical constituents of the PB by various cells such as hepatocytes, bone cells and various tissues for various biochemical and physiological actions in the body system. Excretions of the by-products from unused active ingredients occur through excretory organs of the body (PHC, 2012).

PHARMACOLOGICAL EFFECT

Paxherbal Bitter is a tincture of different herbal ingredients. It promotes blood circulation, prevents kidney stones, helps in digestion and activates bile flow, increase immunity of the body against bacterial and fungal infections. It helps in prevention of diabetes and accelerates body repairs, heal wounds and toothaches (PHC, 2012).

DOSAGE AND CONTRA INDICATIONS

Adults: 20ml/kg which is diluted with 150ml of water before administration. Children: 10ml/kg which is diluted with 75ml of water. It should be stir and drink two times daily and No undue interaction is known yet.

SWEDISH BITTERS

Swedish Bitters is known to be a conventional herbal tonic that helps cure a number of ailments. Originally formulated by Paracelcus. Swedish Bitters was rediscovered during the 18th century by Dr. Urban Hjärne and Dr. Claus Samst, two Swedish medics. Later, an Austrian herbalist Maria Treben strongly promoted it for its wonderful treatment properties. The tonic is available in various formulations in both alcoholic and non-alcoholic versions. Swedish Bitters is known to generally contain rhubarb root, aloe, saffron, camphor, angelica root, zedvoary root, carline thistle root, myrrh, senna leaves and theriac venezia.

USES OF SWEDISH BITTERS

When listing the uses of Swedish Bitters, the list would be quite exhaustive. It can easily be termed as a wonder tonic that heals most ailments you may suffer from. You may use it to clean wounds as an antiseptic, clear away all blemishes or scars from your body, sooth any burns, fight toothache, improve digestion, fight off insomnia and skin allergies, as well as use as a lubricant and treat many more ailments.

Swedish Bitters is extremely helpful for pregnant women and helps fight morning sickness. It is excellent for breast-feeding moms as it works effectively in reducing the inflammation of the nipples. Even people suffering from epilepsy, eye infections, hemorrhoids, frostbites, eye diseases etc have shown great improvement by consuming this tonic.

BENEFITS OF SWEDISH BITTERS

The benefits of Swedish Bitters are plenty. It can be easily prepared at home too and can be stored for a long time without any worries of it getting spoilt. The beauty of this tonic is that the potency increases with time. Swedish Bitters is an effective antiseptic and speeds the healing process by assisting in closing the wounds. On repeated application, you would be able to observe visible changes in the wound. As in Swedish Bitters the herbs are mixed with alcohol it acts as a strong disinfectant by keeping the affected area dry and moisture-free along with combating the infection. It eradicates the toxins and the herbs help in healing naturally. Swedish Bitters is effective against blisters in the mouth too and would help bring down any oral infection. Swedish Bitters is the best possible solution for all stomach ailments. Acidity, gas, cramps, indigestion, bloating etc can all be effectively brought under control by consuming Swedish Bitters. Even for chronic insomnia, it has been observed that people get a restful sleep by consuming the tonic before sleeping.

SIDE-EFFECTS OF SWEDISH BITTERS

In spite of the wonderful results, there may be slight side effects that you may witness. The general side effects that have been reported so far are dehydration, allergy, rashes, cramps or indigestion. Although completely herbal and safe, like all medications it is advisable to first consult your doctor prior to consuming the drug.

YOYO CLEANSER BITTERS

All over the world, the use of organic drugs is becoming increasingly popular. Even in the developed countries, the use of organic products in the therapy of certain diseases is becoming generally acceptable.

Research has now proven that organic drugs are efficacious which allows for such products to be recognized and listed among registered drugs. In Nigeria, it is gradually becoming acceptable that organic drugs can be used side by side with orthodox medicine in the treatment of diseases. So far, all organic drugs in Nigeria are in a way recognized by the national regulatory body (i.e. National Agency for Food and Drugs).

ADMINISTRATION AND CONTROL – (NAFDAC)

Yoyo Cleanser bitters is an organic drug in the class of bitters that was launched into the market by Abllat Company Nigeria Limited. Since its introduction into the Nigerian drug market, it has received wide acceptance and usage by the general population. It will be an understatement to say that it has become a household name. Its acceptability may be attributed to the safety and efficacy in most cases as there has been minimal report of adverse reaction due to its administration.

Yoyo Cleanser Bitters is a bitter in the class of the internationally acclaimed bitters.

COMPOSITION OF YOYO CLEANSER BITTERS

Composition: - (Except ingredients no details mentioned)

1. Aloe Vera

2. Acinos Arvensis

3. Citrus Aurantifolia

4. Chenopodium Murale

5. Cinamomum Aromatiaum / Composition each 5ml contains : -

6. Alhagi Camelorum

7. Cassia Angustifolia

8. Commiphora Myrrha

9. Andrographis Panniculata

10. Picrorhiza Kurroa

11. Tinospora Cordifolia

12. Aloe Barbadens

13. Crocus Sativus

PHARMACOKINETICS

Yoyo bitters rapidly and completely absorbed from the gastro-intestinal tract after oral administration. The phytochmeical ingredients act synergistically to produce its action. Upon sub-chronic administration it increases heamatological parameter and has an LD_{50} of 84.44g/kg body weight (Mendie, 2010).

PHARMACOLOGICAL EFFECT

Indications: -

This Drug is formulated in such a way that the ingredients have a synergistic effect on the management of: -

DIGESTIVE SYSTEM

- It decreases the stomach acidity in cases of ulcer

- It diminishes the irregular production of gastric juice.

- It stimulates the liver to ensure proper and complete digestion

- It helps to digest heavy and fatty food.

CIRCULATORY SYSTEM

- Enhances blood circulation

- Helps to facilitates blood pressure through arteries dilation

- Assists in the elimination of cholesterol, sugar triglycerides,

- Creatine and uric acid

NERVOUS SYSTEM

- Enhances effective function of the secretive glands

- It is beneficial in the treatment of such disorders as insomnia, Stress and depression.

URINARY AND EXCRETORY SYSTEMS

- Facilitates the process of blood purification by the kidneys;

- Helps to dissolve existing kidney stones and to prevent the formation of new ones;

- Prevents Kidney and bladder infections;

- Help to normalize the Operation of the intestine.

ULCERATION

- Inhibits ulceration by eliminating any traces of stored toxins in

- The body system and aid boosting body immunity.

HARDENING OF TISSUES.

- It dissolves any encased toxic materials in the body.

- Enhances cell formation and growth

OVER WEIGHT

- Reduces excess body fat.

- Healthy weight loss

DOSAGE

A maximum adult dose of 30ml/kg thrice daily is recommended.

COMPARATIVE STUDY: -

Similarities

All the herbs used in YOYO are stomachic, carminative & known to tone up the function of Digestive system. The herb "Acinos Arvenis" acting as a Diuratic and Stomachic, is used in YOYO.

All the herb used in Healthy Bitters are also stomachic, carminative & known to tone up the function of Digestive system. The herb Crocus Sativus acting as a diuretic, stomachic and Carminative is used in Healthy Bitters.

Difference / Observation

These type of herbs are not used in YOYO. The herb "Aloe vera" Known to tone up liver function & digestive system, is used in YOYO. No Herb with potent and Anti oxidant. Mild laxative herbs like Cassia Angustifolia and Alhagi Camelorum are use in Healthy Bitters. Along with Aloe vera, the herbs Picrorhiza, Kurroa, Andrographis Panniculata which are known to relieve liver problems used in it. Hence the synergistic action of these herbs makes Healthy Bitters more potent. Anti-Oxidant action owing to Tinospora Cordifolia.

Product Evaluation

The safety and evaluation of the product was conducted by Department of

Pharmacology, College of Medicine, University of Lagos and it was recommended to be safe in experimental animals. Another test was conducted by Multi-Consult Laboratory Limited, Lagos, Nigeria and it showed that the product was sterile and microbiologically fit for human consumption.

Recognition

In April 2010, the product was recognized by the Nigeria Medical Association (NMA) as the NMA Golden Jubilee Official Bitters. In Sept 2010, Yoyo Bitters was given the Health Efficacy Award by the National Post-Graduate Medical College of Nigeria (Faculty of Radiology) in Lagos State University Teaching Hospital.

Conclusion (Yoyo Bitters)

As compare to the formula of YOYO, the formula of healthy Bitters is better in the following respects: -

As the blend of Picrorrhiza Kuroa & Andrographis Panniculata along with

Aloe vera promotes healthy digestion and aiding in condition of sluggish

liver. Healthy Bitter has an efficacy to tone up function of digestive system as well as the liver.

CHAPTER TWO

2.0   Materials and Method

2.1   Materials

2.1.1   Sample material

Yoyo bitters was purchased from a reputable pharmaceutical store opposite university of Benin Teaching Hospital, situated along Ugbowo Lagos road, Ugbowo Benin City, Nigeria. It was bought as a liquid formulation and stored at room temperature (27 ± 2^0C) throughout the period of the experiment.

There include volumetric flask 250ml, conical flask, stopper, water bath (HH-W constant temperature water bath, B. Bram scientific and instrumental company England), Burette, pipette, separation funnel, spectrophoto meter (T70 un/vis spectrophotometer. PG instrument LTD UK) and oven.

2:1:2 **Equipment/Apparatus**

There include volumetric flask 250ml, conical flask, stopper, water bath (HH-W constant temperature water bath, B. Bram scientific and instrumental company England), Burette, pipette, separation funnel, spectrophoto meter (T70 un/vis spectrophotometer. PG Instrument LTD UK), oven.

2:1:3   **Chemical/Reagents**

> For determination of Alcohol content

10ml of 0.05 mol/1potassium dutromate

20ml of 50% sulfuric acid

0.1mol/1 sodium triosulfate

> For determination of total phenol

50ml diethyl ether

Concentrated amylacohol

> For determination of alkaloids

10% acetic acid

Ethanol

Ammonium hydrocide

➢ For determination of Tannin

2ml of 0.1M fecl (non trichloride)

0.1N Hydrochloride acid

0.005M potassium ferrocyamide

➢ For determination of flaunoids

100ml of 80% aqueous methanol

➢ For determination of cynogenic glycoside

20ml of 2.5% NaOH

Silicon oil

8ml of 6N NH_4OH

2ml of 5% Kl

0.02N silver nitrate

Methods

- ### Test Materials

Yoyo bitters was purchased from a reputable pharmaceutical store opposite University of Benin Teaching Hospital, situated along Ugbowo, Lagos road, Benin city, Nigeria. It was bought as a liquid formulation and stored at room temperature ($27\pm2^{0}C$) throughout the period of the experiment.

Solutions

- 0.05 mol/I potassium dichromate (CAUTION- hazardous substance)

- 50% sulfulric acid (CAUTION-highly corrosive)

- 0.5 mol/1kI

- 0.1 mol/1 sodium thiosulfate

- 1% starch solution- made by adding 100mL of boiling water to 1 g of starch powder.

Procedure

1. Pipette 10 ml of bitter into a 250 ml volumetric flask and make up to the mark with water.

2. Place a 5 mL aliquot of the diluted bitter in a conical flask and add 10 mL of 0.05 mol/I potassium

dichromate. Slowly add about 20 mL of 50% sulfuric acid solution to each flask.

3. Stopper each flask loosely and heat in a water bath, at no more than 50°C, for, for at least 60 minutes.

4. Remove from the water bath and add about 10mL of 0.5 mol/1 KI.

5. Titrate the content with 0.1mol/I sodium thiosulfate solution. When the brown colour of the solution gets a green tinge, add a few drops of starch indicator. Continue adding thiosulfate solution until the solution goes a clear, green-blue

colour. This is the endpoint of the titration. Triplicate measurement was performed and the mean computed.

Calculation:

% Alcohol = $\dfrac{(V_2-V_1)* M(S_2O_3{}^{2-})* 0.25*}{M.M_{ethanol}*R* DF}$

Equivalent weight of sample in grammes *100

V_2 = Volume of $S_2O_3{}^{2-}$ solution used for blank

V_1 = Volume of $S_2O_3{}^{2-}$ solution use for sample

M ($S_2O_3{}^{2-}$) = Molar concentration of $S_2O_3{}^{2-}$

0.25 = equivalent of ethanol in mole to 1 mole of $S_2O_3{}^{2-}$

$M.M_{ethanol}$ = molar mass of ethanol

R= ratio of the total extraction volume to the volume used for titration. DF = dilution factor= 25

Determination of total phenols by spectrophotometric method

Total phenol contents in the extract were determined by the modified spetrophotometric method and Onwuka, (2005). The fat free sample was prepared by transferring 5ml odf sample into separating funnel and adding 50ml diethyl ether, shake vigorously and allow to stand. 0.2500g equivalent in ml of the aqueous extract was pipette into 50ml flask, followed by the addition of 10ml of distled water. 2 ml of ammonium hydroxide solution and 5 ml of concentrated amylalcohol were also added. The samples were made up to mark 25ml and colour developed was measured using a spectrophotometer after 30 minutes at 505 nm under room temperature. Triplicate measurement was performed and the mean computed. Total phenolic content were expressed as (g/ 100ml) or (%) tannic acid equivalent.

% Phenols = $\underline{100*C* A_n * V_1}$ (Onwuka, 2005)

$$W * A_5 * V_a$$

Where

A_n = Absorbance of test sample

A_5 = Absorbance of standard solution.

C = Concentration of standard solution

W = Weight of sample used

V_1 = volume of extract

V_a = volume extract analysed

Determination of alkaloids using Harborne (1998) method and Onwuka (2005)

5.0000g of the sample was weighted into a 250 ml beaker and 200 ml of 10%

acetic acid in ethanol added. The beaker was covered and allowed to stand for 4 hours. It was then filtered and the extract concentrated on a water-bath to one-quarter of the original volume. Concentrated ammonium hydroxide was added dropwise to the extract until the precipitate was collected and washed with dilute ammonium hydroxide (2M) and then filtered. The residue if available is the alkaloid which is then dried at $60^{0}C$ in an oven for 30 minutes, cooled and reweighted.

Triplicate measurement was performed and the mean computed.

% alkaloids = $\underline{W_2\text{-}W_1}*\underline{100}$ (Onwuka, 2005)

$$W \qquad 1$$

Where:

W= weight of sample

W1= weight of empty filter paper

W2= weight of paper + precipitate

Determination of Tannin by Van-Burden and Robinson (1981) method.

0.5g equivalent in ml of the aqueous extract was pipette into a 50 ml plastic bottle, 50 ml of distilled water was added and shaken for 1 hour in a mechanical shaker. This was filtered into a 50 ml volumetric flask and made up to the mark. Then 5 ml of the filtrate was pipette out into a test tube and mixed with 2 ml of 0.1M $FeCl_3$ in 0.1N HCl and 0.008M potassium ferrocyanide. The absorbance was measured at 120 nm within 10 minutes. Triplicate Tannin content were expressed as (g/100ml) or (%) tannic aid

$$\%Tannin= \frac{100* C* A_n *V_1}{W * A_s * V_a} \text{ (Onwuka, 2005)}$$

Where:

A_n = Absorbance of test sample

A_s = Absorbance of standard solution

C= Concentration of standard solution

W= Weight of sample used

V_1 = volume of extract

V_a = volume of extract analysed

Determination of Saponins

The method used was described by Obadoni and Ochuko (2001). 20g of each sample in the equivalent volume of liquid sample was put into a conical flask followed by the addition of 100 ml of 20% aqueous ethanol. They were then heated over a hot water bath for 4 hours with continuous stirring at about 55°C. the mixture was filtered and the residue re-extracted with another 200 ml of 20% ethanol. The combined extracts were reduced to 40 ml over water bath at about 90°C. the concentrate was transferred into a 250 ml separatory funnel and 20 ml of diethyl ether added and shaken vigorously. The aqueous layer was recovered while the ether layer was discarded. The purification process was repeated. 60 ml of n-butanol was added. The combined n- butanol extracts were washed twice with 10 ml of 5% aqueous sodium chloride. The remaining solution was heated in a water bath. After evaporation the samples were dried in the oven to a constant weight. Saponin content was calculated as percentage.

Triplicate measurement was performed and the mean computed.

$$\%\text{saponins} = \frac{W_2 - W_1}{W} * \frac{100}{1}$$

Where:

W=weight of sample

W1= weight of empty evaporating dish

W2 = weight of dish + dried sample.

Determination of flavonoids by the method of Boham and Kocipai-Abyazan (2004)

10,0000g in weight of the equivalent volume of liquid sample liquid was extracted repeatedly with 100ml of 80%

aqueous methanol at room temperature. The whole solution was filtered through Whatman filter paper No 42 (125mm).

The filtrate was later transferred into a crucible and evaporated into dryness over a water bath and weighed to a constant weight. Triplicate measurement was performed and the mean computed.

$$\%\text{Flavonoids} = \frac{W_2 - W_1}{W_1} * 100$$

Where:

W= weight of sample

W1 = weight of empty crucible

W2 = weight of crucible + dried sample.

Determination of Cynogenic glycoside (AOAC1984)

Principle

Cyanogenic glycoside are anti-nutrients glycosides that contain the cyanide (-CN) group

Procedure

10,000g equivalent weight of liquid sample is put into 250ml round bottom flask. 200ml of distil water is added and allowed to stand for 2hours (for autolysis to occur). Full distillation is then carried out and 150-170ml of distillate is collected in a 250ml conical flask containing 20ml of 2.5% NaOH. An antifoaming agent (silicon oil or tannic acid) is added before distillation.

To 100ml of the distillate containing glycoside, 8ml of 6N NH_4OH and 2ml of 5% Kl is added, mixed and titrated with 0.02N silver nitrate ($AgNO_3$) using micro-burette against a blank background. Permanent turbidity indicates end point. Triplicate measurement was performed and the mean computed.

Cynogenic glycoside (mg/100g) = $\dfrac{\text{Titre Value ml} *1.08(g) *\text{Extract Volume (ml)})*100}{\text{Aliquot Volume (ml)} * \text{Sample Weight}}$

OR

Cynogenic glycoside (g/100g) or(%) =

$\dfrac{\text{Titre Value ml} *1.08(g) *\text{Extract Volume (ml)})*100}{\text{Aliquot Volume (ml)} * \text{Sample Weight}}$

CHAPTER THREE

RESULT FOR QUANTITATIVE PHYTOCHEMICAL ANALYSIS OF YOYO BITTERS

The quantitative phytochemical analysis of Yoyo bitter and the pharmacological function.

The standard deviation was calculated using Microsoft Excel 2007 and results confirmed using Graph pad statistical Analyzer 2007.

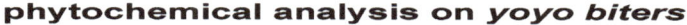

phytochemical analysis on *yoyo biters*

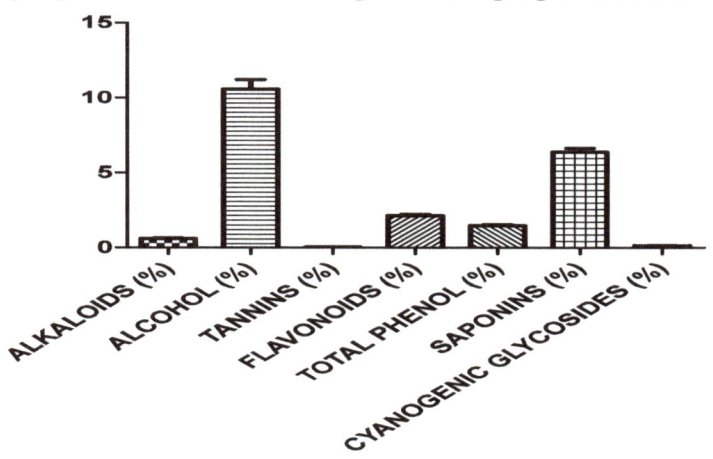

PHYTOCHEMICAL ANALYSIS
OF *Yoyo biters*

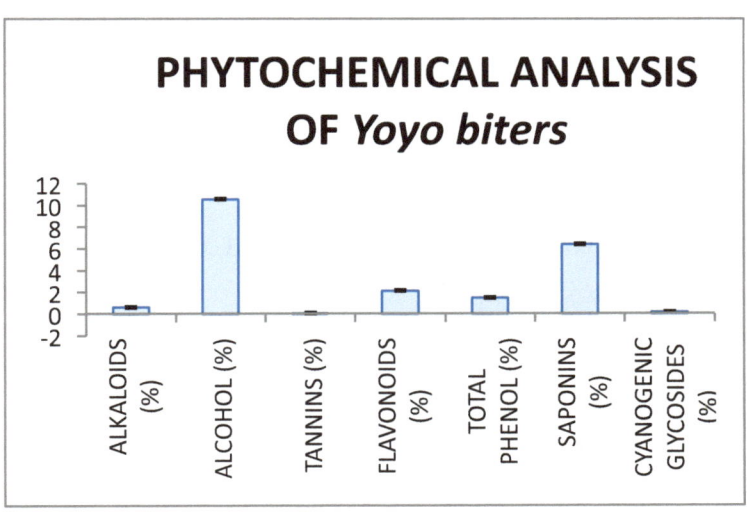

CHAPTER 4

DISCUSSION

All the herbs used in YOYO are stomachic, carminative & known to tone up the function of Digestive system. The herb "Acinos Arvenis" acting as a Diuratic and Stomachic, is used in YOYO.

All the herb used in Healthy Bitters are also stomachic, carminative & known to tone up the function of Digestive system. The herb Crocus Sativus acting as a diuretic, stomachic and Carminative is used in Healthy Bitters.

The inclusion of these ingredients makes the cleanser herbal extremely effective in the gastro-intestinal system, as an anticancer, anti inflammatory and they may be due to the claim about being act as weight loss (Hope; 2009)

Example of the phytochemicals include Alkaloids, Alcohol, Tannins, Flavonoids, Saponins, Total phenol and Glycocides.

Thus phytochemicals varies in percentage in the cleanser herbal remedy. Based on the result of the phytochemical, Alkaloids have low percentage, in the cleanser herbal remedy.

Alcohol has the highest percentage which follows by Saponins then flavonoids and followed by total phenol.

These type of herbs are used in YOYO BITTERS. The herb "Aloe vera" Known to tone up liver function and digestive system, is used in YOYO. No Herb with potent and Anti oxidant. Mild laxative herbs like Cassia Angustifolia and Alhagi Camelorum are use in Healthy Bitters. Along with Aloe vera, the herbs Picrorhiza, Kurroa, Andrographis Panniculata which are known to relieve liver problems used in it. Hence the synergistic action of these herbs makes Healthy Bitters more potent. Anti-oxidant action owing to Tinospora Cordifolia.

Yoyo bitters rapidly and completely absorbed from the gastro-intestinal tract after oral administration. The phytochemical ingredients act synergistically to produce its action. Upon sub-chronic administration it increases heamatological parameter and has an LD_{50} of 84.44g/kg body weight (Mendie, 2010).

This Drug is formulated in such a way that the ingredients have a synergistic effect on the management of: -

DIGESTIVE SYSTEM

- It decreases the stomach acidity in cases of ulcer

- It diminishes the irregular production of gastric juice.

- It stimulates the liver to ensure proper and complete digestion

- It helps to digest heavy and fatty food.

CIRCULATORY SYSTEM

• Enhances blood circulation

• Helps to facilitates blood pressure through arteries dilation

• Assists in the elimination of cholesterol, sugar triglycerides,

• Creatine and uric acid

NERVOUS SYSTEM

• Enhances effective function of the secretive glands

• It is beneficial in the treatment of such disorders as insomnia, Stress and depression.

URINARY AND EXCRETORY SYSTEMS

- Facilitates the process of blood purification by the kidneys;

- Helps to dissolve existing kidney stones and to prevent the formation of new ones;

- Prevents Kidney and bladder infections;

- Help to normalize the Operation of the intestine.

ULCERATION

- Inhibits ulceration by eliminating any traces of stored toxins in

- The body system and aid boosting body immunity.

HARDENING OF TISSUES.

- It dissolves any encased toxic materials in the body.

- Enhances cell formation and growth

OVER WEIGHT

- Reduces excess body fat.

- Healthy weight loss

DOSAGE

A maximum adult dose of 30ml/kg thrice daily is recommended.

CHAPTER 5

CONCLUSION (Yoyo Bitters)

As compare to the formula of YOYO BITTERS, the formula of healthy Bitters is better in the following respects: -

As the blend of Picrorrhiza Kuroa and Andrographis Panniculata along with

Aloe vera promotes healthy digestion and aiding in condition of sluggish liver. Healthy Bitter has an efficacy to tone up function of digestive system as well as the liver.

www.ingramcontent.com/pod-product-compliance
Lightning Source LLC
Chambersburg PA
CBHW040808200526
45159CB00022B/51